It's a
DAD!

*Every man's guide to pregnancy,
birth and becoming a father.*

DEDICATED TO:

The Father of all fathers by whose grace I live

Every man who embraces the awesome privilege
and responsibility of becoming a dad

My two wonderful offspring who have taught
me all I know about fatherhood and inspired me
to put it down on paper

CONTENTS

CHAPTER FOUR:
The Birth

CHAPTER FIVE:
Home Again

CHAPTER SIX:
Dads Matter

CHAPTER ONE:

Becoming DAD

"Dads are most ordinary men turned by love into heroes, adventurers, storytellers, singers of songs."

— Pam Brown

Congratulations! You are about to take on the most important and inspiring role of your life. In the words of Winnie the Pooh, "A grand adventure is about to begin". It started the day your partner announced she was carrying your child. Pregnancy, labour, birth and adjusting to a newborn child is a roller coaster of emotions and changes. Equipping yourself for the ride is one of the greatest gifts you can give your child, your partner and yourself.

Becoming a father is both an incredible privilege and a huge responsibility. As a dad you will be the most influential man in your children's lives. You will be your son's first hero and your daughter's first romance.

This is something worth preparing for, and preparing for well.

This guide will take you through your partner's pregnancy, the birth of your child and the early days of being a father. It will give you invaluable insight into what it takes to be a great dad and show you how to support your partner through her pregnancy and the birth of your child. It will also help you understand and process your own thoughts and feelings about becoming a father.

Becoming a parent is the greatest natural upheaval to your life you will ever experience. It's crazy that we need a licence to drive a car or own a gun but there is no preparation or exam required for the far more complex and important role of being a parent. And most of the available material, courses and interventions for expectant parents is geared towards moms. Yet as the person who will be the most important man in your child's life it's vital that you equip and prepare yourself for the role of dad and partner to the most important woman in your child's life, their mom.

From the moment your partner announced her pregnancy she has most likely been the centre of attention, and when your baby comes they'll both be the centre of attention, not you. On top of this there will be greater demands on your time, energy, money and heart than ever before. Your world is about to change radically and that takes some getting used to. Not much attention is paid to you and how you might be feeling about this whole fatherhood thing, but it's very important to access and deal with what you are experiencing.

As a dad-to-be it's common to feel a wide range of emotions, some very positive, others not so positive. You may feel fear and trepidation, some sadness about losing your freedom, overwhelmed by the responsibility of raising a family, and at the same time joy and happiness. You will have many unspoken questions like, do I have what it takes to be a father? Will I be able to provide? Will my life ever be the same again? When will I have time for golf, sport, friends, myself? Am I ready for this? Why did we do this?!

Here are some of the common fears men experience as fatherhood looms ever closer:

- Fear of not being able to protect and provide for my family.

- Fear of not being able to perform when my partner is in labour.

- Fear of not being able to be there for my child

through death, sickness or accident.

- Fear for my partner's or child's health.

- Fear of not bonding with my newborn child.

- Fear that my relationship will suffer. Will my child be more important to my partner than me, will we have any time together, will we still have a sex life?

- Fear of the whole pregnancy and birth process – the gyni visits, pre-natal classes, labour and birth.

- Fear of not being a good father.

Every one of these fears is common and real. But the truth is you have everything it takes to be a great partner and father. The fact that you are reading this book shows you have the will and desire to get it right. And you will. You won't be perfect but no father is. And that's perfectly okay. Your child doesn't need perfection, he or she just needs you.

Here are seven important things to understand and practise as you prepare for fatherhood:

1. BE CONSCIOUS. Becoming a parent can unlock stuff we never dealt with from our own childhood experiences and trigger emotions that have been buried deep in our psyches. Most of this happens at a subconscious level but often spills over into our moods, actions and responses. This is a time to be very conscious of your feelings and responses and those of your partner.

Whatever you are feeling is real and valid, and deserves to be dealt with. Don't suppress or deny, be very open and honest with yourself about your feelings and take action to deal with them. It may mean going to see a coach or counsellor, having a beer with a close friend or chatting to a mentor or older man.

2. COMMUNICATE. This can never be emphasised enough, particularly to men. Whatever you are feeling, whatever doubts and struggles you have, communicate with your wife. You are partners in this process and being a parent will test this partnership like nothing else. You will naturally have different views and feelings about different aspects of parenthood and that is both healthy and normal. The most effective way to make sure these differences don't cause conflict is open, honest, consistent communication about everything. The more you communicate the easier every aspect of the journey will be for the whole family.

3. WORK ON YOURSELF. Fatherhood is about imparting to our kids all they need for success in life. And we father out of who we are as men. Few men had manhood, masculinity and fatherhood well modeled for them and as a result every man has some degree of woundedness in his heart and psyche that has has carried into adulthood from his own childhood experiences.

There is no greater inspiration for working to get our own lives and hearts whole and free than being a father. We can only give our children what we have inside to give, and chances are that whatever we do have in our hearts we will impart to them in some way. This applies to both the good and the bad. If we have love, joy, peace and goodness in our hearts that's what we will impart to our children. If we have anger, prejudice and a lack of forgiveness in our hearts, that's what we will impart to them.

What incredible motivation to make sure we have the right stuff in our hearts!? Being a father is a parallel journey – learning to be and become a whole man as we raise our daughters to become women and our sons to become men. Most fathers either perpetuate the style of fathering they experienced or work hard at doing the opposite. Conscious fathers do neither – they look at what is best for their children and they do that.

4. TRUST THE PROCESS. As men we often want to fix things, and have everything under control. Fatherhood tests that to the limit. As one man said, "before I had children I had six theories about raising children, now I have six kids and no theories". There will be many times during the pregnancy and birth that you will not be able to step in and "fix it". You will need to trust your partner and the beautiful course of nature.

Even if you don't always have the solution, just be there. Being present and engaged is the greatest gift you can give your loved ones.

5. CONNECT WITH OTHER MEN. The problem with most men is we keep our feelings to ourselves and shoulder the burden of our emotions alone. It is far more healthy and beneficial to be real and honest about what you are feeling and to share it. Millions of men have walked this road and felt the same fears and doubts that you do. Find someone you trust who is a bit further along the fatherhood journey to help you discuss, offload and process what you are going through.Share with other men, read books about other men's experiences, chat about your hopes, dreams and fears.

6. GET INFORMED. As with everything we do in life, the more knowledge and information we have, the better. One of the great benefits of living in the world we do is there is unprecedented access to information. Admittedly, that includes access to misinformation and rubbish too, but we don't have any excuse for being uninformed or under-informed about anything.

Take the time to research and read about pregnancy, birth and being a great dad. Don't just take everything your doctor or clinic says as gospel; check for yourself, ask questions, get different views. Bringing a young life into the world is the most important thing we ever do and it warrants being super-well informed.

7. UNDERSTAND YOUR PARTNER'S JOURNEY.

While you are processing your own emotions and getting ready for your new role your partner will be dealing with some pretty radical changes of her own. Pregnancy is a beautiful and natural process but it does involve some quite significant physical, emotional and hormonal challenges and changes.

Understanding the changes your partner will go through during her pregnancy is crucial to providing her with the support she will need.

Having children is always more difficult than you think and also more rewarding than you can imagine. In almost every decision we make in life it's possible to weigh up the pros and cons and draw up a balance sheet of sorts listing the costs and benefits. Having a child is different because it's impossible to know and understand the incredible value and positives it will bring into your life until it actually happens. Although fatherhood turns life as you know it on its head, it's worth it. All of it.

"Whether your pregnancy was meticulously planned, medically coaxed, or happened by surprise, one thing is certain – your life will never be the same.

– Catherine Jones

CHAPTER TWO:

Pregnancy – a Beautiful Minefield

"Love is all fun and games until someone loses an eye or gets pregnant."

-Jim Cole

Your child's life starts the second your partner falls pregnant, and the best start he or she can have is a happy, healthy, well rested and stress free mom during pregnancy. In more ways than one a happy, healthy mom makes for a happy, healthy baby. The body and mind of a pregnant woman create the environment for the most crucial stage of a child's development. Her emotional state, what she eats and drinks, how healthy and active she is all contribute to the health and development of the baby inside her womb.

Childbirth educator Lauralyn Curtis describes pregnancy beautifully: *"In some cultures, the word for 'pregnant mother' is the same as the word for 'new mother', which essentially translates as Motherbaby:*

implying that whatever affects the mother also affects the baby, both before birth and after birth. You can think of the Motherbaby as a new-born entity who requires a great deal of care, nourishment, kindness and support throughout the slow transition into two separate, distinct beings. She needs to be fed, held, comforted. She needs sleep, support and safety. Most of all, a new-born mother should never be left to cry it out alone. Someone needs to respond to her cries; someone needs to be there to reach out and say 'I know... I know... it's so hard... it feels impossible, and yet I know that you can do it, because you ARE doing it...'"

The experience of being pregnant differs from woman to woman. Some women go through their entire pregnancy with relatively little discomfort (considering the massive physical and hormonal changes involved), whilst others struggle from beginning to end. It's important to understand the changes your partner will be going through and to make life as easy as you can for her (as long as she doesn't take too much advantage!).

There's no way of knowing where your partner will fall on the continuum from hating to loving pregnancy until she is actually experiencing it. But whatever the experience is for her, you are in a better position than anyone to support her through it.

> "It's an established fact.
> Some women can't stand being
> pregnant, getting big and bloated,
> and hauling around a giant
> stomach, and some women, for
> reasons probably understood by
> Darwin, love it."
>
> – Rich Cohen.

Although a mother's emotions don't pass through the placenta, hormones do. A stressed, anxious mom produces stress hormones which are transferred to the baby. By supporting your partner both physically and emotionally, you are helping her mind and body to create the best possible environment for your baby to develop and grow in.

WHAT TO EXPECT

There are two sides to being pregnant. There is the beautiful, wonderful blessing side. The second side - it sucks!"

-Tamar Braxton

There is something truly beautiful about a pregnant woman. The life blossoming inside her reflects in a radiance about her; she is in her prime, literally bursting with life and womanhood. Yet she goes through tremendous physical and hormonal changes which can be very taxing emotionally. Living with a pregnant woman can be a little like walking through a beautiful minefield. Lovely flowers might be blooming all around, the scent and buzz of nature alive in the air, but take one wrong step and you could lose a limb.

The reality is that your partner will experience some quite radical physical changes, and the hormones her body releases will affect her emotional state. She will need you to understand and support her through this beautiful but challenging time.

Here are some of the effects she is likely to experience:

QUEASINESS. Morning sickness is somewhat of a misnomer as nausea and vomiting can strike pregnant women at any time of day. Fortunately, this side effect of pregnancy usually passes by week 12 or so.

BREASTS. Her breasts will grow. That's not an invitation to touch, as appealing as it might be. Her breasts are preparing for breast feeding and can become very tender. Don't be alarmed if late in her pregnancy she starts leaking milk; it's perfectly normal.

EXTRA BLOOD. All the hard work of pregnancy requires more blood vessels and more blood. By the 20th week of pregnancy, the volume of blood in her body will have increased by more than a litre from the time she conceived. All this extra blood can have some strange side effects, including varicose veins, haemorrhoids, and even the famous pregnancy "glow" as she gets more circulation to her skin. Extra blood may also result in nosebleeds and nasal stuffiness as her mucous membranes swell.

FREQUENT URINATION. An increase in blood volume puts more pressure on her kidneys and later in pregnancy the weight of the baby on her bladder increases the pressure even more, making her feel like she always has to go to the toilet.

MOUTH AND TOOTH CHANGES. Her body needs extra calcium for the baby and if it doesn't come from her diet her body will steal it from her bones and teeth. Her gums may also bleed more easily.

FATIGUE, MOODINESS AND FORGETFULNESS. She will experience tiredness and periods of being more emotional than usual. This is caused by a combination of the flood of extra hormones in her system, carrying the extra load and difficulty in sleeping comfortably.

ACHES AND PAINS. During pregnancy, ligaments and tendons throughout her body stretch to accommodate the growing baby and to allow the baby out during labour. This can lead to aches and some pain, particularly in the lower abdomen. She may also experience carpal tunnel syndrome in one or both hands, caused by compression of the nerves that carry signals to the hand and fingers.

SHORTNESS OF BREATH. By the end of her pregnancy, with the baby pressing up against her diaphragm, she may feel as if she can't get enough air.

CONSTIPATION. Caused by pregnancy hormones.

HEARTBURN AND GAS. Most pregnant women experience this in the third trimester. The pressure of the uterus on the stomach, coupled with the relaxation of the valve between the stomach and oesophagus, allows stomach acid to "reflux" into her throat.

LEG CRAMPS. She may experience sudden leg cramps, a feeling that something is crawling on her legs or have an uncontrollable urge to move her legs, particularly at night.

That's quite a list! And all this on top of watching her own body get bigger and bigger, the physical strain of carrying around the extra weight and the emotions that go with bringing another life into the world that will be 100% reliant on her. Makes me glad to be a man!

The bottom line is that your partner needs you during pregnancy. And so does your child. She needs you to understand what she is going through, to be kind, patient, loving and supportive. Be gentle and encouraging, give up your need to be right all the time, listen to her and affirm her feelings.

SEX, DRUGS AND ROCK 'N ROLL

*"Sex is a part of nature.
I go along with nature."*

-Marilyn Monroe

In a healthy pregnancy there is absolutely no danger in having sex at any stage (until her waters break and she goes into labour, that is!). It will also not have any negative effect on your baby. There will be no repressed memories of an ugly, blunt object trying to stab them in the womb requiring extensive therapy later in life. So put your mind at ease.

In fact, because of the physical and emotional benefits and all the positive chemicals released during lovemaking, it is highly recommended. As she gets larger you will need to get very creative and find positions that even the Kama Sutra would struggle to identify.

When it comes to sex, however, an expectant mother's changing body can be the source of a lot of conflict, misunderstanding and confusion for couples. Changes in the desire for sex are common for both men and women during pregnancy. There is no "normal" or standard level of desire or sexual activity for men or women; it differs from man to man and woman to woman.

For some men, seeing a woman carrying their child validates their masculinity and makes them hornier than ever. They find their partner's growing body to be deeply feminine and desirable. Many dads-to-be feel closer to their partner than ever and that closeness can lead to an increase in desire.

For other men pregnancy is a time of reduced sexual desire. Now that she's pregnant her body might seem more functional than sexual. Her growing tummy can make it feel as if there's a third person in the bed, or her leaking breasts may seem rather messy than enticing.

Your partner will also experience a range of feelings about sex during pregnancy. She may feel more connected to you than ever and find the idea of having created a life with you to be wildly erotic. She may be delighted with her curvier body or she may feel large and unattractive. The hormones coursing through her veins can at times enhance desire and at other times quench it. If she experiences bouts of nausea during her first trimester, sex will be the last thing on her mind.

As her partner there are two very important things you can do:

COMMUNICATE: talk openly about how you are feeling, ask her how she is feeling, listen and understand.

AFFIRM HER: with all the physical and emotional changes she is experiencing she will need to hear you tell her you love her and still find her desirable.

Alcohol and smoking are best avoided completely during pregnancy and the best thing you can do to help your wife with this is to join her and encourage her in her abstinence. Don't tell her not to have a drink as you sit sipping a chilled glass of well wooded Chardonnay.

EXERCISE RULES

In a healthy pregnancy there is no problem exercising. In fact, it is highly recommended. On top of all the usual benefits of exercise it can help ease discomfort during pregnancy and will certainly help your partner get back her pre-pregnancy shape after birth.

Walking and swimming are great choices. The key is for her to stay well hydrated, not overheat and avoid anything that could cause her to fall or take a hard knock. Sports such as water skiing or rock climbing, and contact sports such as basketball or soccer are best avoided.

FOOD, CRAVINGS AND AVERSIONS

"By far the most common craving of pregnant women is not to be pregnant."

- Phyllis Diller

It's very important for your partner to eat well during her pregnancy. What she eats directly affects her baby. She will not need to radically increase her food intake as a woman's body makes more efficient use of the energy she gets from food during pregnancy. It's a bit of a myth that she will need to eat for two. The key is for her to eat a variety of foods that are nutrient-dense, such as lean meats, fruits, vegetables and whole grain products, and fewer sweets and treats.

In an ideal world a balanced diet is all she will need but an antenatal vitamin-mineral supplement may be good insurance to make sure she's getting all the nutrients she and the baby need.

She may experience cravings for some foods and strong aversions to others. No one really knows why pregnancy cravings occur. The predominant theory is that they represent some nutrient that the mother may be lacking and the craving is the body's way of asking for what it needs.

High hormone levels present during pregnancy often alter a woman's sense of taste and smell which can make certain foods and odours more enticing. It can also make others more offensive which leads to pregnancy food aversion. Food aversions mostly happen in early pregnancy when they are likely to spark off a bout of morning sickness with nausea and vomiting.

YOUR DEVELOPING BABY

"For you created my inmost being; you knit me together in my mother's womb".

- Psalm 139:13

A baby's brain grows and develops significantly throughout the entire pregnancy, which is why healthy pregnancy habits for all nine months are so important. There is little definitive research on the benefit of stimulating your baby's brain while still in the womb but there is no doubt that playing soothing music, singing and talking to your baby has a positive effect.

Babies start to respond to sound from about 20 weeks. They're aware of noises inside the womb, such as blood gushing, heart pumping and digestion working, as well as outside, such as music. New-born babies are known to respond to sounds and voices they heard whilst in the womb, so the baby definitely has awareness and memory in the later months of pregnancy.

Babies open their eyes in the womb at around 22 weeks. Although their eyesight is still very limited at that stage, they are able to see the bright light of the sun as a warm glow if mom strips off to catch the sun. Babies have a sense of touch and respond to being stimulated within the uterus from about 17 weeks.

There is a definite correlation between a mother's emotional life while pregnant and the emotional predisposition of her child later in life. An anxious mother is more likely to produce an anxious baby. This is because of the stress hormones that pass through the placenta and give the baby a greater physiological propensity for being anxious later in life.

Short-term emotional upsets and quickly resolved anxieties experienced during pregnancy do not harm the baby emotionally but long periods of anxiety and stress can affect the baby adversely. There is also evidence to show that mothers who resented being pregnant and felt no attachment to their babies are more likely to have children with emotional problems. Mothers with less anxious pregnancies and whose babies are wanted and loved have a higher chance of having emotionally healthy children.

All this makes it very important to minimise your

partner's stress and worry during pregnancy by making sure she feels safe and secure; emotionally, physically and financially.

CHAPTER THREE:

Preparing for the Big Event

> *"Birth is the sudden opening of a window, through which you look out upon a stupendous prospect. For what has happened? A miracle. You have exchanged nothing for the possibility of everything."*
>
> *- William MacNeile Dixon*

Giving birth to a child is one of the biggest, most emotional and altogether most mind blowing experiences you and your partner will ever have. It is worth preparing for well as there are no re-runs.

There is no need to fear though. Child-birth is a beautiful and natural process. You can't hurry it and you can't stop it. The truth is it will happen whether you are involved or not. But the great news is that you can make a huge difference as a man to the quality of the birth experience; for yourself, your partner and your baby.

BIRTH PLAN

A very worthwhile exercise is to spend time with your partner preparing a birth plan which records your preferences for the kind of birth you would like to have. There are many things to consider and lots of great templates available, so find and choose one that works for you.

Here are some of the main items to include in the plan:

LABOUR

- Pain relief preferences

- Delivery position options

- Who she wants as birthing partners

- What type of delivery does she want?

- What are her pushing preferences?

- Does she want a mirror to view the birth?

- Does she want the birth to be filmed or photographed?

- What kind of fetal monitoring do you both want?

- What sort of labour props does she want?

- Does she want to wait for her water to break naturally?

- Does she want an episiotomy or natural tear?

AFTER BIRTH

- Does she want to hold your baby skin-to-skin immediately after delivery?

- Do you want to delay clamping and cutting the umbilical cord?

- Do you as the dad want to cut the umbilical cord?

- Do you want to donate your baby's cord blood to a public bank?

- Do you want to store your baby's cord blood in a private bank?

- Would you like to delay newborn procedures such as bathing and measuring for the first hour to give her a chance to feed and bond with your baby?

- Would you like all procedures done and all medications given to baby to be explained to you beforehand?

- If your baby has to be taken for medical treatment,

would you as dad like to go along or stay with your partner?

- Does she plan to exclusively breastfeed the baby while in the hospital or birth centre?

- Would your consent be required to give formula to your baby?

- What are your circumcision preferences if your baby is a boy?

This list is by no means exhaustive so do some research and find a checklist that works for you and your partner. It's a great way of getting to understand all the different options available during and immediately after birth. Obviously in the case of a Caesarean section there are fewer options and variables.

Here are some of the many benefits to preparing a birth plan:

- You will go into the birth well informed and knowing what to expect.

- You will have time to discuss and agree on options in a calm and rational setting (not under pressure during the birth).

- You are less likely to encounter any surprises during

labour and birth.

- It will guide you in your choice of birthing facility and the kind of medical professional you would like in attendance.

Remember that nature may decide not to follow your script perfectly at the time of the birth, so keep an open mind in case things don't go exactly as planned.

Most couples leave everything in the hands of their doctor and the birthing clinic and trust implicitly what they recommend. Researching and preparing a birth plan will empower you to choose both the medical professional and the clinic that best suits the kind of birth you would like to have.

PRACTICAL PREPARATIONS

To make the birth and homecoming of your child as stress free as possible here are some practical things you can do:

- Get ahead on household admin and paying bills so you don't have to worry about that when the baby comes home.

- Pre-register at the hospital or birthing clinic so by the time you arrive all the administration is done.

- Treat your partner to a good spa treatment shortly before the birth. She won't have much time for that for a while.

- Stock up on diapers, wipes and all the baby paraphernalia you will need.

- Make sure your partner has a bag packed with all the clothes and toiletries she will need during her stay at the birth clinic.

- Install the car seat and make sure you know how to use it (practice securing a teddy bear or co-operative pet)

- Get the baby's room ready.

TERMS TO KNOW

THE UTERUS OR WOMB is where the baby grows and lives during pregnancy.

THE CERVIX is the opening (sphincter) that the baby travels through to get out into the world. During pregnancy the cervix is tightly closed to help keep the baby inside the uterus and during childbirth it opens up to allow the baby to pass through the vagina.

DILATION is when the entrance to the cervix opens up to allow the baby to pass through. In early labour the cervix will dilate about 3cm. Full dilation is 10 cm.

WATER BREAKING is when the membrane housing the baby (amniotic sac) ruptures. This happens at the onset of or during labour.
Contractions or surges are when the uterus tightens to push the baby out of the womb.

CROWNING is when the baby's head emerges from the cervix and doesn't slide back again. When this happens the birth is imminent.

BREECH is when the baby is positioned feet down in the womb instead of head first.

THE APGAR SCORE is a method used to quickly summarise the health of new-born children (invented by anesthetist Virginia Apgar in 1952). It evaluates the new-born baby on five simple criteria on a scale from zero to two, then adds the five values to get a score from zero to 10. The five criteria and how they are scored are:

CRITERIA	SCORE OF 0	SCORE OF 1	SCORE OF 2
Appearance	Blue or pale all over	Blue at extremities, body pink	Pink all over
Pulse	Absent	Less than 100 beats per minute	Greater than 100 beats per
Grimace	No response to stimulation	Grimace on stimulation	Cry on stimulation
Activity	None	Some flexion	Flexed arms and legs
Respiration	Absent	Weak, gasping	Strong, lusty cry

TYPES OF BIRTH

"My mother's idea of natural birth was giving birth without makeup."

- Robin Williams

Choosing the kind of birth your partner would like to have is a very personal decision and it is primarily hers to make. Men who want to dictate what kind of birth they would like their partner to have are stepping on very thin ice. Share your preferences by all means but respect that this is her body and she has the final say. There are two basic ways to give birth: a Caesarean section or a vaginal birth. They are two very different experiences and it's worth looking at each in some detail.

Caesarean Section Births

A Caesarean or C-section birth is a fully fledged operation which must be done in a medical facility by a surgeon. An unplanned, emergency C-section may be necessary if problems arise during labour that make continuing with labour dangerous to mom or baby. An elective Caesarean section is one that is scheduled ahead of time by the doctor and mother.

Although more and more moms are choosing in advance to have a C-section the only time it is a medical imperative is when a vaginal birth would put the mom or baby at risk. This is only the case in about one in seven pregnancies. The World Health Organisation estimates that a C-section is beneficial in between 10 and 15 percent of births.

It's very interesting to look at the rates of C-section births in different countries. In the USA approximately one third of all babies are delivered by C-sections, in Finland 16 percent and in the United Kingdom 24 percent. In South African private hospitals the figure is an astonishingly high 76 percent. Most of these C-sections are not a medical necessity.

Here are some of the medical reasons for a scheduled C-section:

- Mom has previously had some other kind of invasive uterine surgery, such as the surgical removal of fibroids.

- She is carrying more than one baby. Some twins can

be delivered vaginally, but most of the time doctors feel more comfortable performing a C-section.

- Your baby is expected to be very large (a condition known as macrosomia).

- The baby is in a breech (bottom first) or transverse (sideways) position.

- The placenta is so low in the uterus that it covers the cervix (placental previa).

- Mom has an obstruction, such as a large fibroid, that would make a vaginal delivery difficult or impossible.

- The baby has a known malformation or abnormality that would make a vaginal birth risky.

- Mom is HIV positive.

In the case of an elective C-section your doctor will schedule it for no earlier than 39 weeks, unless there is a medical reason to do so, in order to make sure the baby is mature enough to be born healthy.

Some of the more common reasons that an emergency C-section may be necessary are:

- Mom's cervix stops dilating or the baby stops moving down the birth canal, and attempts to stimulate contractions to get things moving again haven't worked.

- Your baby's heart rate gives cause for concern and continued labour or induction might put too much strain on the baby.

- The umbilical cord slips through the cervix (a prolapsed cord). If that happens, your baby needs to be delivered immediately because a prolapsed cord can cut off the baby's oxygen supply.

- The placenta starts to separate from the uterine wall (placental abruption), which means the baby won't get enough oxygen unless delivered right away.

Generally, moms choose a C-section for one or more of the following three reasons:

1. The convenience of picking the date and time of delivery.

2. Fear of natural childbirth.

3. The misconception that her vagina will never be the same again.

There is a lot of research that suggests that natural childbirth is beneficial to the baby. It is certainly much easier after birth for the mom as she doesn't have to recover from major abdominal surgery. For example after a C-section mom won't be able to drive for at least three weeks, whereas after natural childbirth she can usually drive the next day.

Natural Birth

In 85% of births natural or vaginal birth is perfectly safe. Even if your partner has previously had a C-section it is quite possible to have a safe vaginal birth – this is called a VBAC (vaginal birth after Ceasarean). When it comes to natural birth there are more options than ever available to moms. The type of birth experience she wants is ultimately a very personal decision. The first choice she needs to make is whether she wants to give birth in a natural home-like setting or in a medical facility with all the conveniences of modern medicine close at hand.

While the vast majority of women in the developed world give birth in a hospital there is a resurgence in the number of women wanting a more natural environment. In the case of a high-risk pregnancy or a VBAC, a fully equipped medical facility is the safest option. In a healthy pregnancy with no complications there are other safe options.

Fortunately, most hospitals have vastly improved the

kind of birthing experience they offer. The days of legs in stirrups in a cold, clinical, brightly lit room are largely over. Hospitals do vary greatly though in the kind of birthing environment and options they provide and it's worth investigating to see what is available.

Many hospitals now offer private rooms where you can go through labour, delivery and recovery all in the same room. Often the dad can stay with mom and baby and the rooms are designed and decorated to simulate a home environment. The other options are a home birth or a birthing centre which may or may not be fully equipped with medical equipment for use in case of emergency.

The important thing is to match your choice of birthing facility to the type of birth you and your partner would like to have.

While very few women choose to give birth at home the number is rising steadily. For a healthy mom with a healthy, normal pregnancy home births are perfectly safe.

Home births are not recommended if:

- Mom has health problems such as diabetes or high blood pressure.

- You are having twins or multiple births Y.

- Your partner wants to attempt a VBAC.

- She has a high-risk pregnancy.

- You are far away from medical support should you need it.

Most women who give birth at home work with a midwife and or doula. When choosing a midwife, ask about her qualifications and experience, how many home births she has attended, and who her backup obstetrician is.

WHO TO HAVE AT THE BIRTH

"If there is one thing you can do RIGHT NOW to ensure your best birth experience, it's this: Choose a care provider who is an EXPERT in the type of birth you are planning. If you are planning a safe, skilled Caesarean birth, you should hire someone who is an expert at Caesarean sections. You wouldn't hire a doctor for a C-section who said, "Well actually I'm not really comfortable with that type of birth, but I'll let you do it if you want, I suppose..." If you're planning a safe, natural, unmedicated birth, you should hire someone who is an EXPERT at supporting natural birth. A doctor with a 30% C-section rate is not a natural birth expert. Neither is a doctor who does routine episiotomies, or doesn't understand how to catch a baby unless mom is laying on her back. A doctor who says "Well, most of my clients do end up choosing an epidural, but if you want to go natural you can do that, I suppose..." is NOT an expert in unmedicated birth. When you find the right care provider, they will understand your birth plan before you even show it to them, because it's what they already do EVERY DAY."

- Lauralyn Curtis

There are two kinds of support your partner will need during birth: medical support and emotional support. Having the right team of people to support both of you during birth will make a massive difference to the kind of experience the two of you will have. Medical support can be provided by a doctor (usually an obstetrician or gynecologist) and/or a midwife. You as dad should be the primary source of emotional support for your partner but it is a great comfort to have the wisdom and experience of a Doula (I'll explain what that is soon) during the birth as well.

When it comes to choosing the medical support you and your partner would like to have at the birth make sure that the type of health care practitioner you decide on matches and supports the kind of birth you would like to have. In a normal healthy pregnancy (which is over 80% of pregnancies) it is not necessary to have a medical doctor present during birth (although it is wise to have a doctor and medical facilities close at hand to assist in the unlikely case of an emergency).

International expert in maternity care and safe birth practices, Doctor Marsden Wagner says that there are, in principle, two approaches to assisting at birth. The first is to "work with the woman to facilitate her own autonomic responses", which he calls humanised birth, and the second is to "override biology and superimpose external control using interventions such as drugs and surgical procedures", which he terms medicalised birth. He believes that *"Having a highly trained obstetrical surgeon attend a normal birth is analogous to having a pediatric surgeon babysit a healthy two-year old."*

It's important to remember that pregnancy is not a health problem or a medical condition; it's as natural as the sun rising and setting, and is a normal, healthy physiological process. If you're looking for a health care practitioner who is more likely to take a holistic approach to the care of your partner during pregnancy, and to see birth as a normal process, intervening only when necessary and not as a matter of routine, a good midwife is the way to go.

"Midwives are the experts in normal pregnancies."

- M. Christina Johnson

Midwives are qualified medical professionals trained specifically to assist during the birth process. Because of their medical knowledge and specific training around childbirth they don't need to have a doctor in attendance unless there are complications during the birth. Midwives see childbirth as a natural occurrence, not a medical event. They place a high degree of importance on prenatal education and developing a strong relationship with their patients. As many midwives say they adopt a "very personalised, high-touch, low-tech form of care".

Recent research shows that women with low-risk pregnancies (85 % of pregnancies) who see midwives throughout their pregnancy and whose deliveries are supervised by a qualified midwife undergo fewer inductions, receive fewer episiotomies, require less anesthesia, have more vaginal births after Ceasareans, are less likely to have a delivery using instruments (such as a vacuum or forceps), heal more quickly and are more satisfied with their experience than those who give birth under a doctor's care.

According to the Midwifery Task Force, the midwives model of care includes:

- Monitoring the physical, psychological, and social well-being of the mother throughout the childbearing cycle

- Providing the mother with individualised education, counselling, and prenatal care, continuous hands-on assistance during labour and delivery, and postpartum support

- Minimising technological interventions

- Identifying and referring women who require obstetrical attention.

> "There's no question that women who deliver with nurse-midwives do just as well as those who use doctors, as long as physicians are available to handle emergencies."
>
> — Kenneth Bell, M.D

In addition to having a midwife in attendance, more and more couples are also choosing to engage the services of a doula to assist them through labour and birth. A doula is a birth attendant trained to provide emotional and practical support to a woman and her partner before, during and after birth. Doulas are there to "mother" the mother. Because of their experience and knowledge of childbirth and their calming presence, they make a significant difference to the quality of the birthing experience whether vaginal or C-section. Doulas are great for you as dad too – they enable you to be the support you need to be without worrying about anything.

"Obstetricians have been taught that pregnancy and labor are disasters waiting to happen which means that OBs tend to use more medical interventions and pay less attention to the emotional concerns of women."

- Bruce Flamm, M.D (Obstetrician)

PAIN RELIEF OPTIONS

Labour and childbirth is a painful experience and women vary in their response to it. Most women need some form of pain relief to help them through the process. Some women are keen to avoid drugs or other medical interventions while others are happy to consider all available options. For a woman having her first baby, the experience of labour (and her reaction to it) is unpredictable so it's a good idea to be aware of the available options for pain relief.

It's important to go into labour with a clear plan about what kind of pain relief your partner wants, but also to be open to change should the need arise. She may start labour with the intention of using only natural pain relief but halfway through active labour start threatening you with your life if you don't immediately get the doctor to give her an epidural. Make sure you have discussed this fully and what the signal is for changing her mind.

It is important to let your partner know that you will support her whatever option she chooses and that there is no shame in wanting pain relief. Again this is not a decision you can make for her.

NON-MEDICAL PAIN RELIEF OPTIONS

Drug-free options will never entirely eliminate pain during childbirth but they can make a significant difference to the level of discomfort experienced during labour.

Here are some ways to prepare:

- Being in good physical condition by exercising gently and regularly throughout pregnancy, avoiding cigarettes and alcohol, and eating a healthy, balanced diet.

- Knowing what to expect during the various stages of labour to help reduce anxiety.

- Breathing techniques can help to 'ride the waves' of each contraction.

- Constant, close support from you her partner (or a trusted friend or loved one) for the duration of labour will reduce anxiety.

- Using distractions like music can help to take her mind off the pain.

- Hot or cold packs, massage, a warm shower or immersion in a warm bath, and keeping active may all be helpful.

The most common non-chemical pain relief option during labour is Transcutaneous Electrical Nerve Stimulation (TENS). This is a technique in which nerves in the lower back are stimulated using a small hand-held device controlled by the woman. It has no known side effects for mother or baby and many women find it helpful either alone or in combination with other methods of pain relief. If you decide to use a TENS device your partner will need to hire one before she goes into labour and practise using it. Usually this form of pain relief is more useful in the earlier stages of labour.

MEDICAL PAIN RELIEF OPTIONS

There are three main medical pain-relieving options for labour:

1. **Nitrous oxide** (also known as laughing gas or "gas and air")

2. **Pethidine**

3. **Epidural**

Nitrous oxide

Nitrous oxide is administered to the mother through a face mask or a tube held in the mouth. It doesn't stop the pain entirely, but takes the edge off the intensity of each contraction. Many women prefer nitrous oxide because it allows them direct control – she can hold the mask herself and take deep breaths whenever she feels the need. Nitrous oxide doesn't interfere with contractions and it doesn't linger in either the mom or baby's body.

Possible problems with using nitrous oxide include:

- Nausea and vomiting.

- Confusion and disorientation.

- Claustrophobic sensations from the face mask.

- Lack of pain relief – in some cases (about one-third of women) nitrous oxide doesn't offer any pain relief at all.

- It's more of an interim solution and not for the whole birth, often used while waiting for an epidural or if you arrive at the facility too late for an epidural.

Pethidine

Pethidine is a strong pain reliever (related to morphine and heroin) which is usually injected intra-muscularly. The effect of pethidine can last anywhere from two to four hours. Because it often leads to nausea, anti-nausea medication is usually administered at the same time.

Possible problems with pethidine for mom include:

- Dizziness and nausea

- Disorientation

- Lack of pain relief in some cases

There is some debate about the effect of pethidine on newborn babies. Potential problems include:

- The baby may struggle to breathe initially at birth. This can be reversed by an injection given to the baby.

- The baby's sucking reflex may also be depressed.

Epidural anaesthesia

Epidural injections are the most effective pain relief available and they allow mom to stay awake and alert during the birth. Epidurals are used for both vaginal births and Caesarean sections. It involves injecting an anesthetic into the lining of the spinal cord through the back which numbs mom from the waist down.

Possible side effects and complications of epidural anaesthesia include:

- Sometimes the numbing effect is not complete and mom may still feel some pain. In this case the procedure will need to be repeated.

- After the epidural has been inserted, mom's blood pressure may drop, leaving her feeling faint and nauseous. This may also cause stress to the baby which is treated by giving intravenous fluid.

- An epidural can cause some muscle weakness in the legs, so women who have had an epidural anaesthetic may be confined to bed for a short while after birth.

- The lack of sensation in the lower body means that mom will not be able to tell when she needs to urinate so a urinary catheter is usually inserted.

- Epidurals can lengthen the second stage of labour.

- Mom may be unable to push effectively due to altered sensation and reduced muscle strength, and baby may have to be delivered by forceps or vacuum cup.

- Some women experience pain or tenderness where the epidural was injected.

An epidural does not:

- Increase the length of the first stage of labour.

- Increase the likelihood of a Caesarean section.

- Cause long-term backache.

Here is an alternative way of looking at the pain of childbirth by a woman who is both an expert in childbirth and a mother herself:

"What if we referred to the sensations of labour with a word other than "PAIN"? The word PAIN is so small and limited. When I stub my toe, I feel pain. When I eat something that gives me gas, I feel pain. I wish I had a better word to describe what it actually FELT like to birth my babies. There was definitely sensation. A LOT of sensation. I could feel it. But it was good. It was OK! I even enjoyed it. It was so primal and sensual. I remember saying at the beginning of a surge, "This one is going to be really big..." and it WAS, but following every wave of labour was a wave of pleasure and relaxation and love. I felt so sexy. I felt so warm and soft and open and flushed with excitement. I guess you could say the pain of childbirth felt really...good. I wish I could invent a new word for it. The closest word I can think of is POWER, but mixed with surrender, sensuality, sexuality, vulnerability and strength. We belittle women and the birth experience when we refer to it with the same word we use for broken bones and bruises. The pain of labour is transcendent."

- Lauralyn Curtis

CHAPTER FOUR:

The Birth

> *"The knowledge about how to give birth is born within every woman: women do not need to be taught how to give birth but rather to have more trust and faith in their own body knowledge."*
>
> — BirthWorks

Giving birth for a woman is probably the most powerful single experience she will ever go through. It touches and taxes every part of her, it is physically hugely demanding, emotionally mind-blowing and spiritually transcendent. Giving birth is visceral, raw and real and at the same time sacred and sublime. As men we cannot claim to understand it, nor will we ever experience anything quite like it, but we do have the privilege of sharing and witnessing it. For us it's a time to be humble and serve.

LABOUR MATTERS

"We have a secret in our culture, it's not that birth is painful, it's that women are strong."

- Laura Stavoe Harm

Labour is the process whereby mom's uterus squeezes her baby out of her womb, down the birth canal, through her vagina and out into the world. There's a reason it's called labour; it takes a tremendous amount of strength and force to push a baby down the birth canal and through the vaginal opening.

It can be challenging for you as dad too. It is difficult to watch your beloved partner experience such pain and discomfort and not be able to make it go away. You will experience a lot of emotions during the process and most likely feel deeply frustrated that you can't do more to alleviate her pain and speed the whole thing up.

It can also be a bit of a minefield for you. Your partner will have moments of extreme discomfort and may be subject to bouts and outbursts of anger and irrationality. Chances are you will be the first in the firing line. Don't argue, defend or take it personally. This is not the time. Deal with whatever she throws your way, no matter how unreasonable it may seem, graciously, lovingly and gently.

A number of key things happen once baby decides it's time to come out and meet the world.

1. The mucous plug which has sealed the entrance to the uterus for the duration of the pregnancy comes free. The plug may come out as one blob-like lump, in several pieces or simply as increased vaginal discharge over a few days. It can be thick, clear or cloudy and it may be pink or tinged with brown or red blood. This normally happens just before labour starts but can happen a few days before.

2. The waters break. This is when the amniotic sac which has been the baby's home for the last nine months ruptures. This normally happens just before or in the early stages of labour. If labour doesn't begin soon after mom's waters break your doctor may want to induce labour as there is a

slight risk of infection. Note that the sac doesn't always rupture naturally and the birth attendant may use a small instrument to open it up. In rare cases baby might be born inside the amniotic sac which is very unusual but quite safe.

3. The uterus tightens to push the baby down and out. This tightening of the uterus is called a contraction or surge and will get stronger and more regular as labour progresses. A contraction happens when the womb (uterus) tightens and then relaxes, and can be painful. If you put your hand on mom's abdomen during a contraction you will feel it getting harder, then softening when the contraction is over.

4. The cervix will thin and start to dilate, making way for baby the to come through.

5. The pressure of the uterus contracting will eventually open the cervix up to 10 cm to allow the baby to pass through.

6. When the cervix is fully dilated baby's head will start to descend, become visible and then push through the vaginal opening.

7. Once the head is out the rest of baby slides out quite quickly.

8. Not long after baby has come out the placenta will be expelled.

There is no standard time frame for labour, it can take hours or over a day, and every woman will experience it differently. It's not always easy to tell when labour has actually started. Physiologically it begins when the cervix starts to dilate but you can't tell from the outside when this has happened. To complicate matters mom will often experience false or practice contractions before the onset of labour called Braxton Hicks contractions.

Braxton Hicks contractions are irregular and short in duration, lasting a few seconds each. Real contractions are regular in duration and frequency. As labour progresses contractions get more intense and last longer. They may start off lasting a few seconds every 10 minutes or so, but every hour they get closer and closer together and last longer.

It's important to track your partner's contractions. When regular contractions start, time them to see how long they last and how far apart they are. The medical personnel will all ask you these questions. "How far apart are they? How long do they last?" Keep a chart.

The only time mom needs to get to the clinic or place where she will be giving birth is when her contractions are strong and regular - two to three within a ten minute period and lasting from 30 seconds to one minute each. At this stage the cervix will have dilated to about 4cm and active labour will have started.

Labour is divided into three distinct stages:

STAGE ONE is made up of early labour and active labour. Early labour begins when the cervix starts dilating. At this point the mucous plug will have come free and mom's waters may or may not have broken. Contractions will become stronger and more regular and the cervix will keep dilating. Up to the first 4cm of dilation mom can still be at home and doing her best to relax and conserve energy. From the onset of labour up to 4cm of dilation can take up to 12 hours although in second and subsequent births it is often quicker. Active labour starts when contractions are strong and regular – three to five minutes apart. This is when mom needs to get to wherever she will be giving birth. At 10cm the cervix is fully dilated and the baby is ready to come out. Active labour usually takes up to six hours but can vary.

STAGE TWO starts when the cervix is fully dilated and mom needs to work with her contractions to push to get baby out. Mom will know she is fully dilated when she feels the urge to go to the toilet along with her contraction. As the baby's head crowns, mom's vagina will be stretched to the limit and may tear (or the medical professional may make an episiotomy cut). If good progress is not made the doctor may assist at this stage with a suction cup or forceps to get baby out. Once baby's head passes through the vaginal opening it all happens very quickly and your newborn will make his or her entry to the real world.

"If you want to know the feeling, just take your bottom lip and pull it over your head."

- Carol Burnett.

STAGE THREE is when the placenta detaches from the uterus and is expelled. This generally happens within 10 to 15 minutes of the birth. Passive delivery of the placenta is when it comes out naturally, active delivery is when the birth attendant assists in getting it out - usually with medication and gentle pulling on the cord.

A doctor may decide to intervene and carry out a C-section if mom or baby is in any danger during stage one or two.

It's very important to remember that labour and child birth is a natural, beautiful process and nature provides women with all the tools they need to get through it. In a healthy pregnancy a safe, warm, comfortable and stress free environment is all that is needed for a woman's mind and body to take control of the birthing process and deliver a healthy, happy baby. The more relaxed and uninterrupted the woman the greater the likelihood of a smooth and complication free birth and the less likely the need will be for medical intervention.

"The knowledge of how to give birth without outside interventions lies deep within each woman. Successful childbirth depends on an acceptance of the process."

- Anonymous

During labour a number of amazing hormones are released which prepare a woman's mind and body for birth. The more relaxed, calm and home-like her environment is, the more readily these hormones will be released and the better the birth process will be. The three most important of these hormones are, Melatonin, Oxytocin and Beta-endorphin.

1. MELATONIN is the hormone that regulates our sleep cycles and induces a state of drowsiness and relaxation. It is best produced in a quiet, warm and dimly lit environment. Melatonin works together with Oxytocin to make the uterus contract during labour.

2. OXYTOCIN is also known as the love hormone because of the role it plays in sexual intimacy, social interaction, bonding and empathy. **Oxytocin plays a number of crucial roles during and immediately after birth:**

- It stimulates strong contractions of the uterus which help to thin and open up the uterus, move the baby down and out of the birth canal, expel the placenta and limit bleeding at the site of the placenta.

- It stimulates the nurturing and maternal instincts of the mother.

- It contributes to the feeling of euphoria and receptiveness that mothers often feel after natural childbirth.

- It assists in the releasing of milk during breastfeeding (the let-down reflex).

Oxytocin has been called the **shy hormone** and needs **certain conditions before it will be released:**

- A sense of security - in people who are scared or distressed, adrenaline surpresses oxytocin.

- Feeling loved.

- Not having to think and process too much

- Being warm and confortable.

- Not been scared or stressed – adrenaline suppresses oxytocin.

- Not being observed, as this heightens anxiety levels.

Low levels of oxytocin during labour can make the birth a lot more difficult by causing contractions to stop or slow and drawing out the labour process.

3. BETA-ENDORPHIN is the body's natural pain killer and plays several key roles:

- Reduces pain during childbirth.

- Regulates the rate of labour.

- Promotes feelings of bondedness between mother and child.

In unmedicated labour the level of beta-endorphin rises steadily throughout labour and birth. Low levels of beta-endorphin make labour a lot more painful and difficult to bear.

One hormone that is definitely not welcome during birth is **adrenaline**. This is the fight or flight hormone which is produced when we feel threatened or anxious. Too much adrenaline can cause labour to slow and even stop. Although during pushing some adrenaline is good and needed.

"Muscles send messages to each other. Clenched fists, a tight mouth, a furrowed brow, all send signals to the birth-passage muscles, the very ones that need to be loosened. Opening up to relax these upper-body parts relaxes the lower ones."

- William and Martha Sears

YOUR ROLE DURING LABOUR AND BIRTH

"You are a birth servant. Do good without show or fuss. If you must take the lead, lead so that the mother is helped, yet still free and in charge. When the baby is born, they will rightly say: 'We did it ourselves!'"

- Tao Te Ching

Men often worry about whether or not they will be able to perform during labour. Most men are also unsure what their role is and what they can do to help. As men we want to fix things, especially when someone we love is in pain or struggling. Whilst you can't stop your partner's discomfort or speed up the process, the good news is that you have a very important role to play during labour and can do a lot to make the experience easier for your partner.

During early labour there is no need for you and your partner to be at the birthing facility. Your role during this time is to keep your partner comfortable and distracted. She will probably be restless and uncomfortable and may want to walk, watch TV, talk or get you to massage her. She also may not want to be touched, so let her set the tone. This phase can take up to 12 hours and can be a mixture of boredom, frustration and discomfort. Just be there for her, listen to her needs and support her emotionally and physically.

Once active labour starts the discomfort will become more intense and you may be on the receiving end of her fraying temper. Go with the flow and do your best to keep her calm and comfortable. Try looking her in the eye and saying, *"You're beautiful, you're strong, you can do this"*. She will either be inspired or punch you.

"The power and intensity of your contractions cannot be stronger than you, because it is you".

Your primary function during active labour and birth is to create the right environment for your partner and nature to work their magic to bring your baby into the world.

The greatest gift you can give her and the most important contribution you can make to a good birth is to support her emotionally and physically so that she will be calm and comfortable and in the right frame of mind for the birth hormones to be released without any hindrance. When all of the birth hormones are present in the right quantities, in a healthy woman without complications the birthing process is able to take place in a smooth and natural way. The kind of environment most conducive to this is very similar to the kind of environment you would like to fall asleep or get romantic in.

"The parallels between making love and giving birth are clear, not only in terms of passion and love, but also because we need essentially the same conditions for both experiences: privacy and safety."

– Sarah Buckley

Here are the keys for creating the right environment for labour:

- Don't rush or hurry her.

- Be gentle and calm at all times.

- Listen to her needs and meet them as far as you are able.

- Don't engage in conversation that will make her think.

- Speak softly and keep the noise levels down.

- Limit the activity in the room.

- Only let people in who are essential.

- Don't be anxious, it's contagious.

- Less is more - trust her and the process.

- Try not to argue or disagree with her (unless completely necessary).

The best births don't need any intervention, just the right environment for mom and baby to do what comes naturally. Birthing women need encouragement to trust their bodies, and to be the stars of their own labours.

"Birth goes best if it is not intruded upon by strange people and strange events. It goes best when a woman feels safe enough and free enough to abandon herself to the process".

- Penny Armstrong and Sheryl Feldman, A Midwife's Story

The ideal birthing environment is:

- Warm.

- Gently lit.

- Quiet.

- Secure.

- Comfortable.

- Predictable – no sudden changes.

Your job is to create that environment. Rub her back, massage her feet, bring her water and snacks, play her favourite music, help her get comfortable, be the love and support she needs.

BIRTHING AIDS

These are some of the things that can help you and your partner during labour:

MUSIC. Music during labour can help your partner relax and deal more effectively with the pain of contractions. Give some thought to your labour playlist. Choose something positive and relaxing that she likes.

FOOD AND DRINK. Women and her birthing partners need nourishment during labour. Bring along some light, tasty snacks and her favourite non-alcoholic drink with some bendy straws to help her drink it.

AROMATHERAPY OILS. Many women enjoy gentle massage, especially in the early stages of labour. Essential oils in the delivery suite can create a relaxing ambience. Check first which oils are safe to use in labour and if the facility is open to you using them.

BIRTHING BALLS. If your partner is planning to use one of these, make sure you get it early and that she practicss using it.

THE ARRIVAL

*"My mother groaned,
my father wept, into the
dangerous world I leapt."*

— William Blake

Once the baby crowns the attending medical practitioner may ask if you would like to touch your baby's head. It's an amazing experience being able to see, touch and experience your baby emerging into the world. At this stage your partner's vagina will be stretched to the absolute limit and it's not uncommon for it to tear a little to allow the baby to pass through. Some doctors prefer to make a small incision called an episiotomy before the vagina tears.

Giving birth is a messy business. You will be amazed at how much stuff comes out of your partner's vagina. First the baby's head emerges, then after several attempts and much pushing the baby suddenly slithers out into the world covered in blood and goo and quite possibly looking decidedly pissed off by the rude eviction from its comfortable digs.

Then the rest of it comes; blood, a strange plastic-like cord which looks patently unhuman attached to a large organ called a placenta which looks like a Texan steak with veins, then more blood and red bits. It's astoundingly messy. But it's awe inspiring. Be ready to be amazed and in awe of your partner.

> "Childbirth changed my perception of my wife. She was now the bloodied special forces soldier who had fought and risked everything for our family."
>
> - Mohsin Hamid

Immediately after the birth mom will release large amounts of oxytocin which will fill her with a sense of love and a strong desire to bond with her new baby. As her partner, nurture and cherish this time. If possible, clear the room of all other people and give your partner and baby time to lie skin on skin.

The greatest need for both mom and baby after birth

is to bond. Even better if you are able to join in. To make this as special and beneficial as possible don't talk a lot or take lots of photos. Maybe get someone else to take pics so you can be deeply involved. Just be together - you, mom and baby, basking in the glory of new life.

There is a chance that mom may be absolutely exhausted and spent, and not be ready to hold or bond with her baby. Don't be alarmed, it is quite normal. Use the opportunity to hold your newborn and allow mom time to rest and recover.

There is no hurry to cut the cord. There is up to 40ml of iron rich blood still available to the baby after the birth and by waiting to cut the cord you will allow baby to receive this. There is no need to bath the baby immediately either. The vernix (that gooey substance that covers a baby when at birth) has important anti-bacterial, cleansing and temperature regulating properties.

CEASAREAN BIRTHS

Giving birth by C-section is a very different experience from a vaginal delivery. Because baby is removed by surgery, it is of necessity a much more clinical procedure, and you and your partner may feel somewhat detached from the actual process of your baby being delivered. Typically you will be allowed to stay with your partner during the procedure and birth but you will have to scrub up and put on operating theatre garb.

This is a summary of what happens during a Caesarean birth:

- Your partner will be given an anesthetic, usually an epidural, which will numb the lower half of her body but leave her awake and alert for the birth. It's rare these days to be given general anesthesia, except in the most extreme emergency situations. If she's already had an epidural for pain relief during labour, it will often be used for the C-section as well.

- A catheter will be inserted into her urethra to drain urine during the procedure.

- An IV will be set up for fluids and medications (if

she doesn't already have one in). Antibiotics will be administered through the IV to help prevent infection after the operation.

- The top section of her pubic hair will be shaved.

- A screen will be raised above your partner's waist so she doesn't have to see the incision being made. You will be allowed to stand by her side on the side of the screen where her head is (not where all the action is taking place).

- Once the anesthesia has taken effect, her belly will be swabbed with an antiseptic, and the doctor will make a small, horizontal incision in the skin above her pubic bone (a "bikini cut").

- The doctor will cut through the underlying tissue, slowly working down to the uterus, separating the abdominal muscles (usually manually rather than cutting through them) and spreading them to expose the uterus.

- Once the uterus is exposed the doctor will make a horizontal cut in the lower section of it. This is called a low-transverse uterine incision. In rare circumstances, the doctor will opt for a vertical or "classical" uterine incision.

- The doctor will then reach in and pull out your baby.

- The cord will be clamped and cut, and you and your partner will have a chance to see your baby briefly before he or she is handed to a pediatrician or nurse.

- While the staff is examining your newborn, the doctor will deliver the placenta and then begin the process of stitching mom up, layer by layer. This usually takes about 30 minutes - longer than the process of taking out the baby.

- After your baby has been examined you and your partner will be able to hold your precious newborn.

After the surgery, mom will be wheeled into a recovery room and closely monitored for a few hours. You and baby will generally be allowed in the recovery room with her and she can start breastfeeding right away. The nurse will remove the IV and urinary catheter within 12 hours of surgery.

The nursing staff will encourage your partner to get out of bed and walk at least a couple of times the day after surgery. The internal stitches used for closing up mom's uterus will dissolve in her body and the stitches or staples used to close her skin will usually be removed three days to a week later. Expect her to stay in the hospital for about three days.

Although a C-section has become a safe and routine procedure it is still major abdominal surgery and riskier than a vaginal delivery. Moms who have C-sections are more likely to have an infection, excessive bleeding, blood clots, more postpartum pain, a longer hospital stay, and a significantly longer recovery period.

Recovery from a C-section will be measured in weeks, not days, so your partner will need help taking care of herself and your new baby. Since she's recovering from major abdominal surgery, her tummy will feel sore for some time. She will need to take it easy and avoid heavy household work or lifting anything heavier than your baby for about eight weeks. She may need prescription painkillers for up to a week after surgery, gradually transitioning to over-the-counter pain relievers.

Breastfeeding can be challenging in the days after a C-section because of the pain from the healing incision. It may be worthwhile seeing a lactation consultant to help with positions that help mom and baby to be comfortable during feeding.

While it's essential for mom to get plenty of rest once you're home, she will also need to get up and walk around regularly. Walking promotes healing and helps prevent complications such as blood clots. In six to eight weeks, she'll be able to start exercising moderately but it will be several months or longer before she's back to her former fit self.

MEETING YOUR CHILD

No matter what anyone tells you, babies are not pretty when they first pop out. So don't feel guilty if you don't feel an immediate bond. When my son Luke was pushed and cajoled out of the warm embrace of his mother's womb I remember being quite horrified at how he looked. He was nothing like the cute, soft, smiling baby boys of diaper-ad fame. He was squashed, blotchy, mottled, covered in goo and had a look of utter dismay and disgust on his face.

As awe inspiring as the whole birth process was, I didn't feel an immediate sense of connection with this strange creature that had just emerged from the depths.

Moms have the advantage of nine months of bonding with their baby in the womb, feeling it moving and growing within them. By the time their little wonder emerges they have already formed a deep bond, and holding their baby in their arms is a natural extension of this process (not to mention the profound relief of having this increasingly sizable stowaway out of their bodies!).

For men the first tangible experience of their offspring is the messy little creature covered in blood and gunk thrust into their arms and it's often more alarming than exciting. Don't worry though because within days or hours you will begin to fall more deeply in love with your child than you ever thought possible.

With the birth of your child will come a greater capacity to love than you ever had before. You can't possibly understand it before becoming a father; it's something that is born in you with the birth of your child. I remember driving in my car with son Luke when he was just a few months old, strapped into his baby seat next to me, with some soppy rock ballad playing, feeling such emotion that tears streamed down my face.

You will soon realise why you need to feel this way because in the first year you will be subjected to things that you would quite simply not be able to deal with if you didn't. You will come into direct contact with all manner of foul liquids, gasses, solids and semi solids, emitted from every exit channel your little bundle of joy possesses. But because of the crazy overwhelming sense of love you feel you will handle it with aplomb!

CHAPTER FIVE:

Home Again

> *"A perfect example of minority rule is a baby in the house."*
>
> — *Milwaukee Journal*

Life will never be the same again. Your time, your space, your money and your wife are not only yours now. And neither is your heart! A small, helpless creature needs you completely and will soon have you wrapped around their tiny finger. They will win your heart, fill you with more joy than you've ever known, make you more vulnerable than you've ever been, give you a greater sense of pride than you've ever had and demand more of you than anyone ever has.

THE EARLY DAYS

After you arrive home with your newborn baby you and your partner will experience a wild cocktail of feelings; elation, uncertainly, protectiveness, pride, fear, responsibility and many others. You will sometimes feel overwhelmed and will be very lucky to escape periods of exhaustion (some babies sleep well and others just don't!). People who say they sleep like a baby usually don't have one.

"There should be a children's song 'If you're happy and you know it, keep it to yourself and let your dad sleep'."

– Jim Gaffigan

It can be a challenging time for a dad and it's possible to feel a bit used and neglected. A lot is demanded of you and not a lot is given in return. Your partner and your child are the centre of attention, you are most likely working hard, sleeping less and having to help out with all kinds of chores around the house. And on top of all that your sex life will not exactly be on fire.

Days three to six after the birth can be particularly challenging. Generally mom is discharged around day three, just around the time that her milk changes from colostrum to normal breast milk. Her breasts may become engorged, latching may be more challenging and her nipples might be sore. Forewarned is forearmed.

Mom will bleed vaginally for about two to three weeks after birth, a bit like an elongated period. This can last for as long as six weeks.

Believe it or not, it's a wonderful time too and it's important to be conscious and aware of the precious times and moments that will come amidst the chaos. The rewards of being a dad far outweigh any sacrifice you need to make in the early days.

"Babies are always more trouble than you thought —and more wonderful."

— Charles Osgood

Here are some valuable tips for these crazy early days:

1. MAKE TIME FOR THE THREE OF YOU. It will take a while for all of you to get into some kind of routine and find your new rhythm. There is great benefit to having family and friends to help out during this time but it is also very important that the three of you make time to bond and nurture your new family unit. Sometimes mom-in-laws, aunts and other family members can invade that sacred space and you need to be assertive in guarding it. It can be a fine line between being gracious and appreciating the help that friends and family give and setting boundaries for your time with mom and child.

2. UNDERSTAND YOUR PARTNER. Your partner will need lots of love and practical support during this time. Help her to rest as much as she can. Consult and consider her before inviting anyone around even though you will want to show your baby off to all and sundry. She will be very tired and the overdose of hormones she will have experienced during birth may leave her feeling a little fragile. If she is breast feeding her body will not be hers (or yours for that matter). She will feel like a food factory and her nipples may become painful and sensitive. What she needs most from you is love, understanding and practical support.

Help as much as you can with household chores.

3. BE GOOD TO YOURSELF. You may feel rejected by your partner at times. Her focus will be very much on her baby and less on you. Remember that the love she feels for her child is completely different to the love she feels for you, so don't get jealous.

4. GET INVOLVED. Some moms get very protective of their babies, even to the exclusion of dad. Psychologists call this "gatekeeping" and it is something to be aware of and deal with lovingly and firmly. It's important that you get involved in all aspects of looking after your baby. The only thing you can't do is breastfeed, but everything else you can. Show your partner that you can handle feeding, burping, bathing, dressing, changing diapers and handling baby in every circumstance. This is great for you and the baby and also for mom's peace of mind. Show her that she has a highly competent partner.

5. GUARD YOUR RELATIONSHIP. Remember to keep communicating. You won't get a lot of time alone and when you do chances are one or both of you will be too tired to talk. Make time to connect, even if it means getting someone to babysit for an hour or two while you do. Share your feelings, your love, doubts, fears and plans.

6. BE INFORMED. Talk, read up on what the experts

say, share with friends and trusted advisors.

7. BUILD A COMMUNITY. Find people in the same stage of life as you. Having a network of people who can help is invaluable.

8. DON'T "BUBBLE WRAP" YOUR CHILD. One of the best pieces of advice I got was that your child comes into your life, you don't come into theirs. Many parents make the mistake of bubble wrapping their newborn child and adjusting their lives too much to create a quiet, sterile environment for them. This is a big mistake. The quicker your newborn gets used to noise, activity and movement, the more adaptable and relaxed he or she will be. By protecting your baby from noise and action you will simply make him or her more sensitive to it, and less tolerant of it. Play music, have friends around, go out, get your child into your routine and he or she will likely become a relaxed and adaptable child.

9. BOND WITH YOUR BABY. Take every opportunity to bond with your child. Hold, touch, nurture, play, bath and spend as much time as you can with him or her. Get involved and get good at all the practical duties of caring for a baby; changing nappies, bathing, feeding, burping. This will help you bond with your baby and help give your wife a break. The deeper your bond with your child when they are young the deeper your bond will be when they are older. And the deeper the bond you have the easier it will be to influence and discipline them in the years when they really need it. Too many fathers try to bond with their children later in their childhood and struggle because they have lost those vital early years of bonding.

10. TRUST YOURSELF. You've got this thing. You love your child and you want the very best for him or her. Listen to the words of Dr Benjamin Spock when he said, *"What good mothers and fathers instinctively feel like doing for their babies is usually best after all"*.

Compared to other mammals newborn human babies are a lot more fragile and vulnerable. They are unable to lift their heads, move about, keep themselves warm or feed themselves. And they need lots of physical touch and nurturing. There are numerous stories of orphaned babies who have been provided with enough food, shelter and warmth at homes that have taken them in, but because they did not receive enough touch and physical contact they failed to grow and thrive, and in some cases became sick and died. Babies need nurture, and the more you as a dad are able to get involved in physically caring for and bonding with your child the better.

"Having children is like living in a frat house – nobody sleeps, everything's broken, and there's a lot of throwing up."

- Ray Romano

SEX AGAIN

"Amnesia: The condition that enables a woman who has gone through labor to have sex again."

- Joyce Armor

The time it takes to resume lovemaking after the birth of your child varies greatly from couple to couple. Some people start as early as a few weeks, others take a bit longer. After a healthy natural birth there is no stipulated time period to wait. As long as she doesn't feel any discomfort there is no physical reason to keep from making love. Lovemaking should be physically comfortable for your partner by the six week mark. The same applies after a C-section.

The challenge is often more emotional and psychological than physical. There are a lot of things that will make your partner feel less than sexy. To start with she may feel self-conscious about how she looks after all her body has just been through. And with nurturing a young child, tender breasts constantly being sucked on and all the mess and fuss around baby's toilet and eating practices, sex may well be the last thing on her mind.

She is also likely to be tired and have some physical discomfort. You on the other hand have probably had less sex in the last six months than you have had since you and your partner got together, and are raring to go.

Finding time and space for romance and lovemaking can also be a huge challenge. Interruptions by baby crying or simply the fear or anticipation of an interruption can make it hard to get into the mood. Chances are when baby is asleep, either you or your partner will also want to sleep. Yes, this is a time when sleeping can be preferable to sex. I bet you never thought that would ever happen!

It's very important for both of you to be open and honest about how you feel and what you want. Be loving and caring with each other during this period; talk, share, express, understand, empathise. Your needs may differ greatly at this time and if you don't talk about your feelings and expectations it can lead to deep frustrations and real relationship challenges.

Men are able to put things in a box and compartmentalise, for women everything is inter-related. We can have an argument and immediately have sex, or come home from a bad day with a headache and have sex. Women generally need to feel loved and desirable before they can get in the mood. They also respond much better when the environment is conducive and there has been a loving build up to your advances. Even more so now that she is caring for a young child.

Approach sex gently and lovingly, be seductive, start with a back rub or foot massage. She will probably need more than usual to get her in the mood. The general rule is that sex will happen again when she feels sexy again. And the person who has the greatest influence on how sexy she feels is you.

"The difference between sex and death is that with death you can do it alone and no one is going to make fun of you".

– Woody Allen

Don't demand; make her feel feminine, loved and desirable. Help her be a mom by being a dad. Assist with making her life easier in practical ways, show that you see her as a woman and not just a mom. And very soon your sex life will be back on track.

POST-NATAL DEPRESSION

It is normal for a woman to experience mood changes, irritability and weepiness after giving birth. These symptoms are known as the "baby blues" and they usually clear up within a few weeks. However, if these feelings persist it could be the more serious condition known as postnatal depression (PND).

Unlike the baby blues, PND is an illness that is not likely to get better quickly or clear up without help. The sooner you and your partner recognise it and get the support that you need, the less likely it is to become a severe or long-term problem.

About one in eight women experience some level of post-natal depression. It normally starts within the first six weeks of giving birth but can take up to a year to appear. Some women don't recognise they have postnatal depression or they choose to ignore their symptoms because they're afraid of being seen as a bad mother.

Women are more likely to be vulnerable to PND if they have challenges in their life such as money or relationship problems.

Common symptoms of PND are feelings of:

- Sadness

- Inability to enjoy anything

- Fatigue and lack of energy

- Sense of hopeless

- Guilt

- Lack of appetite

- Tearfulness

- Generalised anxiety

Most moms have at least one of these feelings some of the time in the first few months after giving birth and it's normal for her to have good and bad days. But if your partner is feeling these symptoms most of the time and they don't get better, she could have PND.

No one really knows why some women get PND and others don't but it is caused by a combination of hormonal changes, psychological adjustment to motherhood and fatigue.

Additional contributing factors may include:

- A history of depression

- Lack of support

- No family or friends living nearby

- Money, work, health or relationship problems

- Difficult labour

- Premature or unwell baby

- Difficulty in breastfeeding

- Sad memories stirred up by baby's birth

The best natural way to avoid or overcome PND is:

- Lots of rest

- Good diet

- Exercise

- Minimise stress

- Develop a good network of people to talk to, help out and "normaliae" her experience (what she is going through is not abnormal and experienced by many)

Although mild PND can usually be dealt with by self-help strategies, social support and a bit of therapy, more severe PND may need medication. Normally, antidepressants will be prescribed to try and balance brain chemicals.

BREASTFEEDING

Whether or not to breastfeed and for how long is a personal decision. It is however highly recommended for the many benefits it offers your baby. The World Health Organisation recommends exclusive breastfeeding for the first six months, then gradually introducing other nutritious foods supplemented with breastfeeding for up to two years. Breast milk has the ideal mix of nutrients for your child to flourish and thrive as well as antibodies to fend off infections. Babies fed on infant formula have a higher risk of developing allergies, asthma and a range of different infections.

The first milk produced by mom is called colostrum and it is the most nutritious and beneficial for the baby. Mom starts producing colostrum during late pregnancy and continues through the early days of breastfeeding. Colostrum is yellow to orange in colour and thick and sticky. It is low in fat, and high in carbohydrates, protein, and antibodies to help keep your baby healthy. It is extremely easy to digest, and is therefore the perfect first food for your baby. It is low in volume but high in concentrated nutrition for the newborn.

Colostrum has a laxative effect, helping baby to

pass his early stools, which aids in the excretion of excess bilirubin and helps prevent jaundice. The concentration of immune factors is much higher in colostrum than in mature milk. Colostrum also contains high concentrations of leukocytes, protective white cells which can destroy disease-causing bacteria and viruses.

The colostrum gradually changes to mature milk during the first two weeks after birth. This milk is thinner and whiter in colour. During this transition, the concentration of the antibodies in mom's milk decreases, but her milk volume greatly increases. The disease-fighting properties of human milk do not disappear with the colostrum. In fact, as long as your baby receives your milk, he will receive immunological protection against many different viruses and bacteria.

In the first few days it is important to breastfeed your newborn at least eight to twelve times each 24 hours. This allows your baby to get all the benefits of the colostrum and also stimulates production of a plentiful supply of mature milk. Frequent breastfeeding also helps prevent engorgement.

Latching is when the baby has the mom's breast firmly in its mouth and is able to suck and extract milk freely and comfortably. Sometimes babies struggle to latch at first but normally with a bit of patience and perseverance and the guidance of a doula or midwife, mom and baby get it right. Latching and breastfeeding should be comfortable, and if it isn't it could be useful to enlist the services of a lactation consultant.

The action of baby suckling sends a message to mom's brain to release oxytocin which stimulates the release of milk. This is called the "let-down" reflex and is the key to successful breastfeeding. Without a good let-down baby will only receive a small amount of milk and may not grow at a healthy pace or may become frustrated and refuse to breastfeed.

Let-down can also be triggered by mom hearing her baby cry, when it's getting close to feeding time, during a warm shower, or during sexual activity. Let-down can lead to leaking or spraying milk and sometimes menstrual-type cramping especially in the early weeks following delivery.

Breastfeeding can be lonely for a mom in the beginning as it can mean hours away from other people, alone with her baby. It's obviously not something you as a dad can do but **there are a number of things you can do to make it easier for mom:**

- Make sure she has water on hand all the time. Breastfeeding leaves mom very thirsty as her body needs a lot of extra fluids to produce milk. It's a real nuisance for her to get up and fetch anything while the baby is latched on.

- Make sure there are readily available snacks for her - breastfeeding burns a lot of extra calories.

- Know where each of her breastfeeding tools are and be ready to bring them to her at a moment's notice. This includes items such as nursing pillows, nipple cream, gel packs from the freezer, burp cloths, etc. Try and make it so she doesn't need to get up out of her seat for any reason.

- Prepare the breast pump. Pumping milk is probably the least desirable aspect of breastfeeding and you can make life easier for her by cleaning and preparing the pump for her.

- If you aren't able to keep her company while she is breastfeeding make sure she has something to keep her entertained and her mind occupied while she does; books, magazines or charged iPad.

- Get a lot more involved in household chores.

- Encourage her and voice your appreciation for what she is doing. She is likely to be emotional and exhausted and words and acts of encouragement will mean the world to her (even if she doesn't always show it).

- Give her massages and foot rubs.

- Help create calm space for her by keeping other children or pets happily occupied.

- Simply ask her what she needs. Sometimes just you asking is all she really needs.

Okay now you've earned some serious brownie points!

HELPING YOUR BABY DEVELOP

At birth a baby's brain is about 25% of the size of a normal adult brain. By the age of two years his brain will have grown to about 75% of its adult size. This huge brain growth in the first two years makes proper brain stimulation critically important. During this time billions of neuro connections and pathways are made. Optimum stimulation will ensure that your child's brain is activated to reach full potential.

The three absolutely essential keys for ensuring your child's brain develops to its full potential are:

1. STIMULATION THROUGH ALL FIVE SENSES – touch, sight, sound, smell and taste. This will ensure that your child's brain develops to its full capacity.

2. CONSTANT LOVE AND POSITIVE PHYSICAL AND EMOTIONAL INTERACTION.
This will ensure that the neurological pathways that your child develops are emotionally positive and anxiety free.

3. THE RIGHT NUTRITION INTAKE which will ensure the biological building blocks are in place for optimal development.

The best thing you can do is expose your baby to a variety of experiences and activities - without overwhelming her. **Some great activities in the first weeks after birth are:**

- A baby mobile or flashcards for visual stimulation

- A variety of soothing music

- Reading to your baby. Even at this young age, a newborn will enjoy the closeness of being held and the changing tone of your voice as you read.

- Placing your baby on his stomach for a few minutes each day. This allows him to work on gross motor skills which helps to develop his brain as well.

As your baby grows out of the newborn stage introduce more brain-boosting activities such as:

- Playing different styles of music – from classical to rock n' roll. Not too loud.

- Expose your baby to various textures, colours, sights, and sounds.

- Walks outside and visiting different environments

- A variety of toys, interesting baby board books, and even a baby DVD occasionally.

- Spend plenty of one-on-one time with your baby. Talk to him, sing to him, cuddle him like there's no tomorrow.

Let your baby set the pace, they also need lots of rest.

Don't forget, even if you can't afford fancy flash cards or toys, what's most important is that you spend time with your baby. Your presence matters far more than your presents.

CHAPTER SIX:

Dads Matter

> *"A good father is one of the most unsung, unpraised, unnoticed, and yet one of the most valuable assets in our society."*
>
> — Billy Graham

As a dad you will be the most influential and important man in your child's life. You will be their first, most important experience of who and what a man is. What you expose your children to, and what you teach them through your life, words, actions and interactions will impart to them their very sense of self, the inner fabric that will equip them for confidence and success or fear and failure. The words you share with them in their formative years will become their inner voice as adults.

What a beautiful responsibility!

But being a great father doesn't just happen. It takes

a deliberate commitment and consistent action. It cannot be outsourced or delegated; it must be handled personally. Just as a safe can only be opened by the key specifically designed for it, you as a father hold the key to unlock the potential in your child's life.

Here is a story from my own life which bears out how important we as dads are, quoted from **"DAD – The Power and Beauty of Authentic Fatherhood"**

"A year after my divorce, my son Luke decided to come and live with me. At the age of 12 he was a big, strong boy, tall and solidly built. He played rugby, loved riding motor bikes and was a real boy in every way. Yet I also noticed a tenderness and vulnerability in him. More than that, there was a cry, a yearning for masculine nurture. For several weeks after moving in with me, Luke would creep into my bed late at night and just hold on to me tightly. It's hard to explain what passed between us during those prolonged, poignant hugs, but it was profound and beautiful.

I didn't have to say anything; he was drawing substance from me, almost by osmosis. I was his rock, his anchor. I was the source of masculinity and strength for his developing manhood. No matter what I was experiencing inside, no matter what challenges I was facing, I was Luke's dad and he needed me. He had questions that I needed to answer. His young developing masculine soul needed to draw from a man and that man was me, his father.

This was a revelation to me. I realised how much my son needed me, and the impact that I as a father would have on him – for good or bad. I realised that there was a window of opportunity for me to give Luke what he needed and I realised that my willingness and ability to do this would quite possibly be the single biggest influence on his development as a man.

Fatherhood matters deeply, profoundly and undeniably. Any man who becomes a father needs to take this responsibility-laced privilege very seriously. And this applies equally to girls and boys. The questions that my daughter Blythe needed me to answer differed slightly from Luke's but she needed my presence, love and consistent input just as much as her brother did."

Being the most important man in someone's life is a privilege that comes with profound responsibilities. Your children will come to you to answer the deepest questions of their hearts. Throughout their developing years they will ask you a thousand times and in a thousand different ways to answer key questions about themselves that no-one else can answer quite like you can. Questions about their identity, value and validity.

Your son will want to know what it means to be a man and whether he has what it takes. Your daughter will want to know if she is worth fighting for, if you delight in her. Answer well and you will lay an unshakeable foundation for your children's emotional well-being and character. Answer badly or don't answer at all and you will wound them and quite possibly set them up for a lifetime of emotional struggle.

Every father influences the lives of his children forever. That's a given. Whether this impact is for good or for harm is the choice every father has to make.

The wonderful thing about being a dad is that we all get to be a hero. Of course, this means that we have to live up to some pretty high expectations. But that's okay, because every dad has it in him to be a hero to his children. And if we get it right we leave our children with a priceless gift. Impressed into their psyche and souls is the knowledge of a man as a strong, loving sanctuary, a place where there is safety and fun and affirmation.

And they will live their lives out of this reservoir of grace and strength. Our sons are more likely to grow up honourable men, treating women with respect and caring for their own families. Our daughters are more likely to grow up as women of stature, making good choices and building strong families of their own.

The world is crying out for men who will step up to the plate and be great fathers. This is your opportunity to be that dad.

THE FIVE COMMITMENTS OF GREAT DADS

Here are five commitments that will help you be an excellent dad.

COMMITMENT ONE:
Look in the Mirror

"The quality of what we impart to our kids is determined by the quality of our own inner lives."

- Craig Wilkinson

None of us arrived at adulthood unscathed by our childhood. We are all driven in some way by emotional forces from childhood experiences, good or bad, and the beliefs formed in response to those experiences.

The more conscious we are of the forces and beliefs we have carried into adulthood and which drive us as men, the more able we are to deal with them.

Being unconscious of childhood wounds means we are likely to be driven by the negative emotions and beliefs they instilled in us, and to pass these on to our children. Unresolved pain from the past is pain we are condemned to repeat, often at the expense of our children.

"Every boy in his journey to become a man takes an arrow in the center of his heart, in the place of his strength. Because this wound is very rarely discussed, and even more rarely healed, every man carries a wound. And the wound is most often given by his father."

– John Elldredge

Commit yourself to being fully conscious, to breaking any destructive emotional cycles, and to dealing with any baggage you may have brought into adulthood and fatherhood. Being a great dad is a parallel journey – becoming a whole man as you raise your children to become whole and healthy adults.

Work hard at being the type of man you want your son to become, and your daughter to marry.

COMMITMENT TWO:
Call out your Child's Identity

"We don't write the script for our children's lives, we help them read the script that's already written on their souls."

-Craig Wilkinson

The second commitment is to discover and call out the unique identity of your child. To be truly seen is one of the great cries of every heart. Make it your goal to be the first man who truly sees your son or daughter. William Shakespeare said that "It is a wise father that knows his own child".

A good father makes it a mission to discover the essence of his son or his daughter. He hears and sees. He listens to his children's words, their body language, their behaviour, what their eyes and hearts are saying. He knows them. He knows what makes his daughter's heart come alive, what her favourite colour is, her fears, passions, likes, dislikes. He knows what excites his son, what will make him get up early in the morning raring to go.

A father who does this refuses to dictate a life script for his children but helps them to discover the life story already written in their souls. He sees what is already there. He calls to the man inside the boy and the woman inside the girl and says, "Come out, you have a role to play. Come out, you are good and worthy and the world needs what you have to offer. Come out and be fully you, fully alive".

You can only do this by investing a lot of time engaging with your children, consistently, deeply and without distractions.

COMMITMENT THREE:
Validate your Child

"My father gave me the greatest gift anyone could give another person, he believed in me."

- Jim Valvano

Men doubt they have what it takes to be a man, women wonder if they have anything worthwhile to offer the world. Every one of us needs to know that our life matters, that we count, that who we are is okay and good. And every one of us at some stage looked to our fathers to confirm and affirm this.

Great fathers validate their children from a very young age. Their children know they are worthy, that their life counts. They know they have what it takes, that they have something great to offer the world. This comes from affirming not just what your children do, but who they are. The message you need to give your child is; you matter, you are wanted, you are deeply loved, I delight in you.

And you need to give them this message in a thousand

different ways; by your words of affirmation, your gentle touch, your look, your smile, your time. The blessing of validation from you their father will remain as a cloak of affirmation wrapped around your son or daughter long after you have passed on.

COMMITMENT FOUR:
Create a Sanctuary for your Child

"Every father is the architect of his home life."

- Reed Markham

The fourth commitment of great dads is to create a sanctuary in which their children can flourish; physically, emotionally and spiritually. The environment in which our children grow up determines whether they will thrive or merely survive. And as fathers we play a primary role in creating this environment.

Strong, loving, present dads create an atmosphere of warmth, safety and joy in which their children flourish. Angry, abusive fathers create a fearful atmosphere laced with dread in which their children retreat into themselves and their rooms. Absent dads leave a sad vacuum in which their children are forced to find their way without his wisdom and strength.

As fathers we have the ability and the responsibility to create an environment which will nourish and protect our sons and daughters and enable them to thrive. The environment that we create has physical, emotional and spiritual elements, all of which are vitally important. Just as a gardener tends to his nursery to make sure that the conditions are ideally suited to each tree that he plants, so we as fathers need to tend to the environment in which our children live.

To carry the gardener metaphor further, every seed of a particular species of tree that is planted has the same innate potential, but the extent to which each one reaches this potential is determined by the conditions in which it grows. The soil in which it is planted, the water and nourishment it receives, the amount of sunlight it gets and the extent to which it is protected from extreme elements determines how much of its potential will unfold. Trees growing in a poor environment may be strong and resilient (if they survive), but they will also be stunted and fall short of their intended height and strength. As fathers it is our responsibility to create an environment in which our children will grow to their full potential.

Sigmund Freud said that he cannot think of any need in childhood as strong as the need for a father's protection. The children of great dads feel safe. They know masculinity as a place of refuge, safety and consistency. They see their fathers as strong, gentle and present.

Create the right physical and emotional environment for your children by nurturing, protecting and providing for them.

COMMITMENT FIVE:
Equip your Child for Life

"The ultimate goal of parenthood is to equip your children so that they don't need you."

- Craig Wilkinson

The last commitment of great dads is to equip their children for life. The ultimate reward of parenthood, if you get it right, is that your children will always want you. As fathers we are there for our children; they are not there for us. As an involved father you will receive immeasurable joy and fulfilment from fathering your children, but your primary role is to give to them, not receive from them.

"Oh the places you'll go!
There is fun to be done!
There are points to be scored.
There are games to be won.
And the magical things you can
do with that ball will make you
the winning-est winner of all."

– Dr Seuss

Equipping your children for life starts with imparting the life skills and emotional intelligence they need to succeed. Poet and priest, George Herbert said that one father is more than a hundred schoolmasters. Great dads do not leave the education of their kids to peers or the media, they become the principal in their children's school of life.

Equipping your children for life also requires discipline. Set clear, fair and consistent boundaries for your children. Teach them discipline and respect. Remember that being a friend to your children comes a distant second to being their father. Be less concerned with being popular than with doing what's right for your kids.

The final key to equipping your children for life is to model the way for them. Make your life an attractive example of what you want your children to learn and be. Your life speaks far more eloquently than your words.

Ultimately your children learn from your way, not what you say.

A FINAL WORD

"Father! To God himself we cannot give a holier name."

— William Wordsworth

You have it in in you to be an extraordinary father. If you consciously and intentionally embrace these five commitments, you will lay the foundation for your children to build their own great lives. As someone so powerfully said "Succeed as a man and the effect may be felt for your lifetime, succeed as a father and the effect will be felt for generations".

The two most important words in a father's lexicon are: "BE THERE".

Be there physically.
Be there emotionally.
Be there when they need to talk.
Be there for the events that matter to them.
Be there when they reach important milestones.
Be there when they are glad, mad, sad or scared.

BE THERE.

You will impact the lives of your children deeply and forever.

The quality of this impact is in **your hands.**

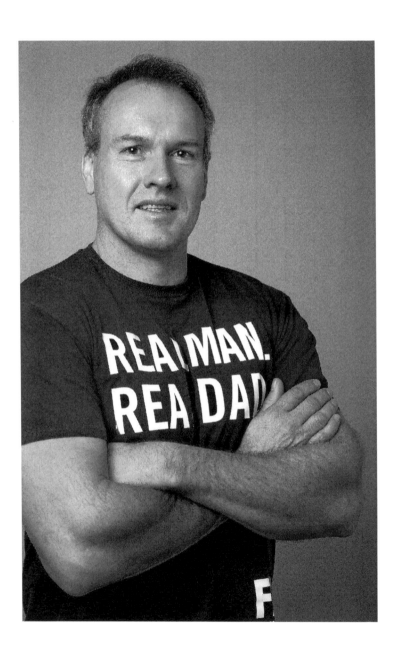

ABOUT THE AUTHOR

Craig Wilkinson lives in Cape Town, South Africa with his wife Martinique and his two children Luke and Blythe.

He is the author of *"DAD – The Power and Beauty of Authentic Fatherhood"* and the online course, *"The Dad Journey"*. Both can be found at **www.thedadbook.co.za**

Craig is a sought after speaker and spoke at **TEDx** Cape Town on the topic of masculinity and fatherhood, see **http://goo.gl/fUFQCJ**

He has worked extensively in the Non Profit sector in the areas of experiential education, socio-economic development and the development of men and fathers as well as a consultant to the corporate sector in strategy and human resource development.

An avid hiker and mountain biker Craig has a passion for the restoration of men to true masculinity and authentic fatherhood. He is the founder of *Father a Nation (FAN)*, an NPO which restores and equips men to be great fathers. He believes that if we can heal men we can heal the world. Some of the work of FAN can be seen at **www.fatheranation.co.za**

You can contact Craig at **craig@fatheranation.co.za**

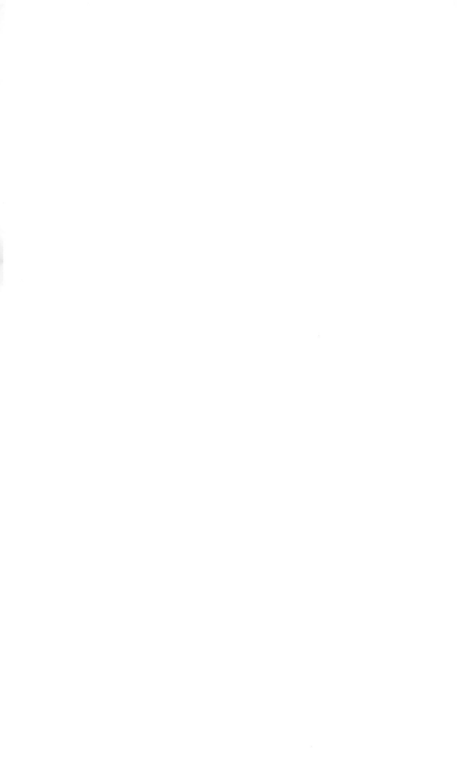

25828190R00081

Printed in Great Britain
by Amazon